DECHAMBEAU'S REVOLUTION:

A New Era in Golf

George G.Porter

De Chambeau's Revolution

All rights reserved. No part of this publication may be reproduced, distributed, or transmitted in any form or by any means, including photocopying, recording, or other electronic or mechanical methods, without the prior written permission of the publisher, except in the case of brief quotations embodied in critical reviews and certain other noncommercial uses permitted by copyright law.

Copyright © 2024 by George G. Porter

TABLE OF CONTENTS

INTRODUCTION

CHAPTER 1: DECHAMBEAU'S EARLY DAYS

CHAPTER 2: THE SCIENCE OF SWING:

CHAPTER 3:THE RISE OF A NEW ERA

3.1: Breaking the Mould:

3.2: DeChambeau's early successes and the golf world's reaction:

CHAPTER 4: THE BIRTH OF A MOVEMENT

De Chambeau's Revolution

4.1: The Trailblazer

CHAPTER 5: THE SCIENCE BEHIND THE SWING

5.1: Unlocking the Secrets of Ball Flight

CHAPTER 6: THE ART OF INNOVATION

6.1: DeChambeau's Approach to Equipment and Technology

CHAPTER 7: MAJOR VICTORIES

7.1: The Impact on the Golf World

CHAPTER 8: OVERCOMING CRITICISM:

8.1: DeChambeau and the Media

CHAPTER 9: THE FUTURE OF GOLF

9.1: A New Generation

CHAPTER 10: THE EVOLUTION OF GOLF:

10.1: A Lasting Impact

CHAPTER 11: BEYOND THE FAIRWAY

CONCLUSION

INTRODUCTION

In the sport of golf, tradition and convention have long been the guiding forces. For over a century, the game has been played with a familiar rhythm: a gentle swing, a precise putt, and a deep respect for the game's timeless principles. But in recent years, a quiet revolution has been brewing. A new generation of golfers, led by the unorthodox and innovative Bryson DeChambeau, has been challenging the status quo and redefining the boundaries of what is possible on the course.

Bryson DeChambeau's rise to the top of the golf world has been nothing short of meteoric. With his

De Chambeau's Revolution

unconventional swing, his reliance on data and analytics, and his fearless approach to innovation, DeChambeau has become a lightning rod for attention and controversy. But beyond the headlines and the hype, DeChambeau's story is one of dedication, perseverance, and a passion for the game that is inspiring a new generation of golfers.

Join us on a journey into the new era of golf, where convention meets innovation and the possibilities are endless.

CHAPTER 1: DECHAMBEAU'S EARLY DAYS

The unconventional beginnings

Bryson DeChambeau's journey to the top of the golf world began in a humble garage in Southern California. As a young boy, DeChambeau would spend hours in his parents' garage, swinging a makeshift club and dreaming of greatness. His father, Jon DeChambeau, a golf enthusiast himself, encouraged his son's passion and began teaching him the fundamentals of the game.

But from the start, DeChambeau's approach was different. While other junior golfers were honing their swings on the driving range, DeChambeau was in his garage, experimenting with unusual grips and unorthodox techniques. He was fascinated by the science of the swing and spent hours studying the movements of the club and the ball.

De Chambeau's Revolution

As he grew older, DeChambeau's passion for innovation only intensified. He began working with his coach, Mike Schy, to develop a swing that was uniquely his own—a swing that blended power, precision, and a dash of creativity. Together, they explored the boundaries of what was possible, experimenting with new techniques and technologies that would eventually become the hallmark of DeChambeau's game.

Early influences

DeChambeau's early days were also shaped by a range of influences beyond golf. He was a curious and introspective child, fascinated by science, mathematics, and philosophy. He devoured books on physics and engineering and spent hours building models and experimenting with new ideas.

These influences would eventually shape DeChambeau's approach to golf, as he sought to apply the principles of science and innovation to his game. But for now, they simply fueled his creativity and his passion for exploration—qualities that would serve him well as he embarked on his journey to the top of the golf world.

CHAPTER 2: THE SCIENCE OF SWING:

Bryson DeChambeau's rise to the top of the golf world was fueled by a revolutionary approach to the game—an approach that blended traditional skill with cutting-edge science and analytics. At the heart of DeChambeau's game was a deep understanding of the physics and biomechanics of the swing, honed through countless hours of research and experimentation.

De Chambeau's Revolution

Data-Driven Insights

DeChambeau's journey into the science of swing began with a simple question: What makes a great golf swing? To find the answer, he turned to data and analytics, working with a team of experts to develop a sophisticated system for tracking and analysing his swing.

Using high-speed cameras, motion sensors, and advanced software, DeChambeau was able to capture detailed data on every aspect of his swing, from the angle of his clubface to the rotation of his hips. He then used this data to identify areas for improvement, fine-tune his technique, and test new approaches.

Biomechanics and Ball Flight

De Chambeau's Revolution

DeChambeau's work in biomechanics and ball flight was particularly groundbreaking. By studying the intricate relationships between clubhead speed, launch angle, and spin rate, he was able to optimise his swing for maximum distance and accuracy.

He also explored the role of the body's core muscles in generating power and stability, incorporating exercises like planks and rotational drills into his training routine.

Geeky Golf

DeChambeau's use of data and analytics earned him the nickname Golf's Mad Scientist, a label he embraced with pride. His geeky approach to the game inspired a new generation of golfers to explore the science of swing, and his innovative methods sparked a wider conversation about the role of technology in golf.

CHAPTER 3: THE RISE OF A NEW ERA

How Bryson DeChambeau is revolutionising golf

Golf has long been a game steeped in tradition, where players adhered to time-honoured techniques and strategies. However, with the arrival of Bryson DeChambeau, the sport is witnessing a seismic shift. DeChambeau's unorthodox approach, fueled by data-driven insights and a relentless pursuit of innovation, is redefining the boundaries of what's possible on the course.

De Chambeau's Revolution

The Birth of a New Paradigm

DeChambeau's rise to prominence marks a significant turning point in golf's history. His maiden major victory at the 2020 US Open was a watershed moment, signalling the dawn of a new era where science and technology converge with raw talent. This fusion has enabled DeChambeau to rewrite the rules of golf, pushing the limits of distance, accuracy, and overall performance.

Key Factors Driving the New Era

Data-Driven Decision Making: DeChambeau's reliance on data analytics has transformed his approach to the game. By leveraging advanced statistics and machine learning algorithms, he gains valuable insights into course management, swing optimisation, and strategy.

Innovative Swing Techniques: DeChambeau's single-plane swing, inspired by the legendary Moe Norman, has become a hallmark of his game. This unique approach, combined with his exceptional strength and flexibility, allows him to generate unprecedented power and precision.

Fitness and Conditioning: DeChambeau's dedication to physical training has raised the bar for golfers worldwide. His regimen, which includes a focus on strength, flexibility, and endurance, has enabled him to maintain a level of consistency and durability throughout the season.

De Chambeau's Revolution

Mental Toughness and Resilience: DeChambeau's mental game is a key factor in his success. His ability to remain focused, adapt to pressure, and bounce back from setbacks has become a model for aspiring golfers.

The Impact on the Golf World

DeChambeau's influence extends far beyond his own achievements. His pioneering approach has inspired a new generation of golfers to embrace innovation and challenge conventional wisdom. As a result, the sport is witnessing a shift towards:

Increased Emphasis on Fitness and Conditioning: Golfers are now recognising the importance of physical training in enhancing performance and extending their careers.

De Chambeau's Revolution

Greater Adoption of Data Analytics: The use of data-driven insights is becoming more widespread.

3.1: Breaking the Mould:

Bryson DeChambeau's rise to the top of the golf world was not without its challenges. As a pioneer of a new approach, he faced scepticism, criticism, and even ridicule from some quarters. However, DeChambeau remained undeterred, driven by a fierce determination to succeed and a willingness to challenge the status quo.

Confronting Convention

From his early days as a junior golfer, DeChambeau was always willing to think outside the box. He rejected the traditional teaching methods and instead sought out his

De Chambeau's Revolution

own unique approach, blending science, technology, and innovation.

As he entered the professional ranks, DeChambeau's unconventional style raised eyebrows. His single-plane swing, his reliance on data analytics, and his intense focus on physical conditioning set him apart from his peers.

Overcoming Scepticism

Despite his early successes, DeChambeau faced a chorus of doubters. Critics questioned his technique, his temperament, and even his commitment to the game. However, DeChambeau remained resolute, using the scepticism as fuel to drive his progress.

De Chambeau's Revolution

Through sheer force of will and an unwavering belief in his approach, DeChambeau slowly began to win over the doubters. His victories, his dedication, and his passion for innovation eventually silenced the critics and earned him a new level of respect.

Paving the way

DeChambeau's willingness to break the mould has paved the way for a new generation of golfers. His innovative approach has inspired others to challenge convention and explore new possibilities.

As the golf world continues to evolve, DeChambeau remains at the forefront, a beacon of innovation and a testament to the power of determination and creativity.

De Chambeau's Revolution

3.2: DeChambeau's early successes and the golf world's reaction:

Bryson DeChambeau's early career was marked by a series of impressive victories and a growing sense of unease among the golf establishment. As he began to make his mark on the sport, DeChambeau faced a mix of reactions, from admiration and curiosity to scepticism and even outright hostility.

Early Triumphs

DeChambeau's first major victory came in 2015 at the DAP Championship, a (link unavailable) tour event. This was followed by a string of successes, including wins at the 2016 DAP Championship and the 2017 John Deere Classic.

De Chambeau's Revolution

As DeChambeau's career gained momentum, the golf world began to take notice. His unique approach, his intensity, and his unwavering commitment to his craft sparked a range of reactions.

Reactions from the Golf World

Some hailed DeChambeau as a visionary, a trailblazer who was pushing the boundaries of what was possible in golf. Others were more sceptical, questioning his unorthodox technique and his reliance on data analytics.

The media was fascinated by DeChambeau's story, with many outlets featuring him in prominent profiles and interviews. Fans were drawn to his charismatic personality and his willingness to challenge convention.

De Chambeau's Revolution

However, not everyone was a fan. Some critics saw DeChambeau as a maverick, a rebel who was disrupting the traditional order of the game. Others questioned his temperament, his sportsmanship, and even his commitment to the values of golf.

The Backlash

As DeChambeau's profile grew, so did the backlash. Some of his fellow players began to question his approach, with a few even suggesting that he was "ruining" the game.

The media, too, began to scrutinise DeChambeau more closely, with some outlets focusing on his perceived flaws and controversies.

Despite the criticism, DeChambeau remained resolute.

CHAPTER 4: THE BIRTH OF A MOVEMENT

Bryson DeChambeau's early successes and his willingness to challenge convention sparked a growing

De Chambeau's Revolution

sense of excitement and curiosity among golfers and fans. As his profile grew, DeChambeau became a magnet for like-minded individuals who shared his passion for innovation and his commitment to pushing the boundaries of what was possible.

A New Generation of Golfers

DeChambeau's influence extended far beyond his own achievements. He inspired a new generation of golfers to embrace innovation, to experiment with new techniques, and to explore the possibilities of data analytics and technology.

Young golfers like Matthew Wolff, Collin Morikawa, and Viktor Hovland began to follow in DeChambeau's footsteps, blending traditional skill with modern innovation.

De Chambeau's Revolution

The Rise of the Golf Nerd

DeChambeau's geeky approach to golf—his love of data, his fascination with physics, and his enthusiasm for technology—helped to spawn a new breed of golf nerds.

These individuals, who combined a passion for golf with a love of science and innovation, began to reshape the sport, introducing new ideas, new techniques, and new technologies that transformed the game.

A Growing Community

As DeChambeau's movement gained momentum, a growing community of like-minded individuals began to

De Chambeau's Revolution

coalesce around him. This community, comprising golfers, coaches, analysts, and innovators, shared a common goal: to push the boundaries of what was possible in golf.

Through social media, online forums, and specialised websites, this community began to connect, share ideas, and collaborate on new projects.

The Future of Golf

DeChambeau's movement marked a significant turning point in the history of golf. As the sport continued to evolve, it was clear that the future would belong to those who were willing to innovate, to experiment, and to push the boundaries of what was possible.

De Chambeau's Revolution

4.1: The Trailblazer

Bryson DeChambeau's impact on golf extends far beyond his own achievements. He is a trailblazer, a pioneer who has opened up new possibilities for the sport.

Paving the way

DeChambeau's willingness to challenge convention and embrace innovation has paved the way for others to follow. His success has inspired a new generation of golfers to think outside the box, to experiment with new techniques, and to explore the possibilities of data analytics and technology.

Breaking down barriers

De Chambeau's Revolution

DeChambeau's trailblazing approach has helped to break down barriers in golf, challenging traditional notions of what is possible and expanding the boundaries of the sport.

He has shown that golf is not just a game of tradition and convention, but also a sport that can be shaped and transformed by innovation and creativity.

A New Era of Golf

DeChambeau's influence has helped usher in a new era of golf, an era characterised by innovation, experimentation, and a willingness to push the boundaries of what is possible.

De Chambeau's Revolution

As the sport continues to evolve, DeChambeau remains at the forefront, a trailblazer who continues to inspire and innovate.

Leaving a legacy

DeChambeau's legacy extends far beyond his own achievements. He has inspired a new generation of golfers, and his influence will be felt for years to come.

As a trailblazer, DeChambeau has left an indelible mark on the sport, a mark that will continue to shape and transform golf for generations to come.

CHAPTER 5: THE SCIENCE BEHIND THE SWING

Bryson DeChambeau's swing is a marvel of modern golf, a blend of traditional technique and cutting-edge science. But what makes his swing so unique? And how does he use science to gain a competitive edge?

The Physics of the Swing

DeChambeau's swing is governed by the laws of physics, particularly the principles of motion, energy, and momentum. By understanding these principles, DeChambeau is able to optimise his swing for maximum power and accuracy.

De Chambeau's Revolution

Biomechanics and Movement Patterns

DeChambeau's swing is also influenced by biomechanics, the study of the structure and function of living organisms. By analysing his movement patterns and muscle activity, DeChambeau is able to identify areas for improvement and optimise his technique.

Data-Driven Insights

DeChambeau uses data analytics to gain a deeper understanding of his swing, tracking metrics such as clubhead speed, ball flight, and swing plane. This data provides valuable insights that help him refine his technique and make adjustments.

The role of technology

De Chambeau's Revolution

Technology plays a critical role in DeChambeau's swing, from the advanced materials used in his clubs to the sophisticated software used to analyse his swing. By leveraging technology, DeChambeau is able to gain a competitive edge and stay ahead of the curve.

The Science of Swing Optimisation

DeChambeau's swing optimization is a continuous process driven by a desire to improve and innovate. By combining physics, biomechanics, data analytics, and technology, DeChambeau is able to create a swing that is both powerful and precise.

The Future of Golf

De Chambeau's Revolution

As golf continues to evolve, the science behind the swing will play an increasingly important role. DeChambeau's approach represents the future of golf, a future where science and technology combine to create a new era of innovation and excellence.

5.1: Unlocking the Secrets of Ball Flight

Bryson DeChambeau's work with biomechanics and ball flight has been a game-changer for his golf game. By understanding the intricate relationships between his body, the club, and the ball, DeChambeau has been able to optimise his swing for maximum performance.

Biomechanics and the Golf Swing

De Chambeau's Revolution

Biomechanics plays a critical role in the golf swing, influencing everything from clubhead speed to ball flight. DeChambeau works closely with biomechanics experts to analyse his swing, identify areas for improvement, and optimise his technique.

Ball Flight Analysis

DeChambeau uses advanced ball flight analysis to gain a deeper understanding of his swing. By tracking metrics such as launch angle, spin rate, and carry distance, DeChambeau is able to fine-tune his technique and make adjustments.

The Role of 3D Motion Capture

De Chambeau's Revolution

DeChambeau uses 3D motion capture technology to analyse his swing, providing a detailed breakdown of his biomechanics and movement patterns. This technology helps DeChambeau identify areas for improvement and optimise his technique.

Working with Ball Flight Experts

DeChambeau collaborates with ball flight experts to gain a deeper understanding of the golf ball's behaviour in flight. By analysing data and testing different variables, DeChambeau is able to optimise his swing for maximum performance.

The Science of Clubhead Speed

De Chambeau's Revolution

Clubhead speed is a critical factor in ball flight, influencing everything from distance to accuracy. DeChambeau works closely with biomechanics experts to optimise his clubhead speed, using techniques such as strength training and swing analysis.

The Future of Ball Flight Analysis

As technology continues to evolve, ball-flight analysis will play an increasingly important role in golf. DeChambeau's work in this area represents the future of golf, a future where science and technology combine to create a new era of innovation and excellence.

CHAPTER 6: THE ART OF INNOVATION

Bryson DeChambeau's approach to golf is a masterclass in innovation. He has revolutionised the sport by combining traditional techniques with cutting-edge science and technology.

Thinking outside the box

DeChambeau's innovative approach is characterised by a willingness to think outside the box. He challenges conventional wisdom and explores new possibilities, often combining seemingly unrelated ideas to create something entirely new.

The power of experimentation

De Chambeau's Revolution

Experimentation is a key component of DeChambeau's innovative approach. He continually tests new techniques, technologies, and equipment, always seeking ways to improve and refine his game.

Collaboration and knowledge sharing

DeChambeau collaborates with experts from a range of fields, from biomechanics to materials science. By sharing knowledge and ideas, he is able to stay ahead of the curve and identify new opportunities for innovation.

The Importance of Failure

De Chambeau's Revolution

DeChambeau views failure as an essential part of the innovative process. He embraces failure as a learning opportunity, using it to refine and improve his approach.

The Future of Golf

DeChambeau's innovative approach has transformed the sport of golf, inspiring a new generation of golfers to think creatively and push the boundaries of what is possible.

The Art of Innovation in Action

DeChambeau's innovative approach is evident in every aspect of his game, from his use of advanced analytics to his experimentation with new equipment and techniques.

By combining art and science, creativity and technology, DeChambeau has created a new paradigm for golf, one that is characterised by innovation, experimentation, and a willingness to challenge convention.

6.1: DeChambeau's Approach to Equipment and Technology

The Tech-Savvy Golfer

Bryson DeChambeau's approach to equipment and technology is a key component of his innovative approach to golf.

Customisation and Innovation

De Chambeau's Revolution

DeChambeau works closely with equipment manufacturers to design and develop customised clubs and balls that meet his specific needs.

Advanced Materials and Manufacturing

DeChambeau is fascinated by the potential of advanced materials and manufacturing techniques to transform golf equipment.

3D Printing and Prototyping

DeChambeau uses 3D printing and prototyping to test new equipment designs and iterate on existing ones.

De Chambeau's Revolution

Data-Driven Decision Making

DeChambeau uses data analytics to inform his equipment choices, tracking metrics such as ball flight, swing speed, and launch angle.

The Role of Simulation and Modelling

DeChambeau uses simulation and modelling software to test and optimise his equipment, simulating different scenarios and conditions to find the perfect setup.

Collaboration with Technology Experts

De Chambeau's Revolution

DeChambeau collaborates with technology experts, including engineers and data scientists, to stay ahead of the curve and identify new opportunities for innovation.

The Future of Golf Equipment

DeChambeau's approach to equipment and technology is transforming the sport of golf, inspiring new innovations and advancements that will shape the future of the game.

By combining cutting-edge technology with a willingness to experiment and innovate, DeChambeau is redefining what is possible in golf.

CHAPTER 7: MAJOR VICTORIES

Bryson DeChambeau's innovative approach to golf has led to a string of major victories, cementing his status as one of the sport's top players.

2019 US Open

DeChambeau's first major victory came at the 2019 US Open, where he held off a strong field to win by six strokes.

De Chambeau's Revolution

2020 Rocket Mortgage Classic

DeChambeau's second major victory came at the 2020 Rocket Mortgage Classic, where he carded a 23-under-par total to win by three strokes.

2020 US Open (Winged Foot)

DeChambeau's most dominant major victory came at the 2020 US Open at Winged Foot, where he carded a six-under-par total to win by six strokes.

2021 Arnold Palmer Invitational

De Chambeau's Revolution

DeChambeau's fourth major victory came at the 2021 Arnold Palmer Invitational, where he carded a 12-under-par total to win by one stroke.

Major Championships: A Timeline

2019 US Open: Won by six strokes

2020 Rocket Mortgage Classic: Won by three strokes

2020 US Open (Winged Foot): Won by six strokes

2021 Arnold Palmer Invitational: Won by one stroke

DeChambeau's Major Victories: A Closer Look

Each of DeChambeau's major victories has showcased his innovative approach to golf, from his use of

De Chambeau's Revolution

advanced analytics to his willingness to experiment with new equipment and techniques.

By combining cutting-edge technology with a fierce competitive spirit, DeChambeau has become one of the sport's most dominant players, with a string of major victories that will be remembered for years to come.

7.1: The Impact on the Golf World

Bryson DeChambeau's innovative approach to golf has sent shockwaves through the sport, inspiring a new generation of golfers and challenging traditional notions of what is possible.

A Changing of the Guard

De Chambeau's Revolution

DeChambeau's rise to prominence marks a changing of the guard in golf as a new generation of players who are more analytical and tech-savvy take centre stage.

Inspiring a New Generation

DeChambeau's success has inspired a new generation of golfers to embrace innovation and experimentation, from amateurs to professionals.

Challenging Traditional Notions

DeChambeau's approach has challenged traditional notions of golf, from the importance of physical strength to the role of technology in the sport.

De Chambeau's Revolution

Transforming the sport

DeChambeau's impact on golf extends beyond his own achievements, transforming the sport in ways that will be felt for years to come.

The Future of Golf

As golf continues to evolve, DeChambeau's innovative approach will play a central role in shaping the sport's future, inspiring new generations of golfers and challenging traditional notions of what is possible.

The DeChambeau Effect

De Chambeau's Revolution

The "DeChambeau Effect" has been felt across the golf world, inspiring a new wave of innovation and experimentation that will transform the sport for years to come.

By combining cutting-edge technology with a fierce competitive spirit, DeChambeau has become a trailblazer for golf, opening up new possibilities and inspiring a new generation of golfers to follow in his footsteps.

CHAPTER 8: OVERCOMING CRITICISM:

Bryson DeChambeau's innovative approach to golf has not been without its critics. From traditionalists who question his unorthodox methods to fans who doubt his ability to adapt, DeChambeau has faced his fair share of criticism.

De Chambeau's Revolution

Dealing with Doubt

DeChambeau has learned to deal with doubters and critics, using their scepticism as fuel to drive his success.

Staying Focused

Despite the criticism, DeChambeau has remained focused on his goals, refusing to let the opinions of others derail his progress.

Building Resilience

De Chambeau's Revolution

DeChambeau's experiences have taught him the importance of resilience—learning to bounce back from setbacks and stay motivated in the face of adversity.

Proving the critics wrong

DeChambeau's success has proven his critics wrong, silencing the doubters and validating his innovative approach.

Turning Criticism into Motivation

DeChambeau has learned to turn criticism into motivation, using the scepticism of others to drive his success.

The Power of Self-Belief

De Chambeau's Revolution

DeChambeau's self-belief has been a key factor in his ability to overcome criticism, staying true to himself and his vision for the game.

By overcoming criticism and staying true to himself, DeChambeau has emerged as a role model for golfers and non-golfers alike, inspiring others to embrace innovation and experimentation.

8.1: DeChambeau and the Media

Bryson DeChambeau's innovative approach to golf has made him a media sensation, with journalists and commentators fascinated by his unique blend of science and skill.

Media Frenzy

DeChambeau's rise to prominence has been accompanied by a media frenzy, with reporters and camera crews eager to capture his every move.

The Mad Scientist of Golf

De Chambeau's Revolution

DeChambeau's analytical approach has led to him being dubbed the "mad scientist" of golf, a nickname that reflects his unconventional approach to the sport.

Profile pieces and interviews

DeChambeau has been the subject of numerous profile pieces and interviews, with journalists seeking to understand the man behind the method.

The Role of Social Media

Social media has played a key role in DeChambeau's media presence, with millions of followers hanging on his every word and move.

Controversy and Criticism

De Chambeau's Revolution

DeChambeau's media presence has not been without controversy, with some journalists and commentators criticising his approach and questioning his commitment to the sport.

Setting the record straight

DeChambeau has used the media to set the record straight, addressing criticism and misconceptions about his approach and his personality.

A Media Icon

DeChambeau's media presence has cemented his status as a golf icon, with millions of fans around the world following his every move and hanging on to his every word.

De Chambeau's Revolution

By embracing the media and using it to his advantage, DeChambeau has become a household name, inspiring a new generation of golfers and non-golfers alike.

CHAPTER 9: THE FUTURE OF GOLF

Bryson DeChambeau's innovative approach to golf has opened up new possibilities for the sport, inspiring a new generation of golfers and challenging traditional notions of what is possible.

A New Era for Golf

DeChambeau's success marks the beginning of a new era for golf, an era characterised by innovation, experimentation, and a willingness to challenge convention.

De Chambeau's Revolution

The Role of Technology

Technology will play an increasingly important role in golf's future, from advanced analytics to cutting-edge equipment and training methods.

The Next Generation of Golfers

DeChambeau's influence can be seen in the next generation of golfers, who are already embracing innovation and experimentation in their approach to the sport.

Golf's Growing Popularity

De Chambeau's Revolution

Golf's popularity is on the rise, thanks in part to DeChambeau's influence and the sport's increasing appeal to a younger, more diverse audience.

The Evolution of Golf Course Design

Golf course design will evolve to accommodate DeChambeau's innovative approach, with courses that challenge and reward players who think creatively and strategically.

The Future of Golf: A Predictive Model

DeChambeau's use of data analytics and predictive modelling will become increasingly influential in golf, allowing players to optimise their performance and gain a competitive edge.

De Chambeau's Revolution

By combining innovation, experimentation, and a willingness to challenge convention, DeChambeau is helping to shape the future of golf, inspiring a new generation of golfers, and cementing his status as a true pioneer in the sport.

9.1: A New Generation

Bryson DeChambeau's impact on golf extends far beyond his own achievements, inspiring a new generation of golfers to embrace innovation and experimentation.

The DeChambeau Effect

De Chambeau's Revolution

The DeChambeau Effect has been felt across the golf world, with young golfers everywhere seeking to emulate his approach and attitude.

A New Breed of Golfer

DeChambeau's influence has given rise to a new breed of golfer, one that is more analytical, more experimental, and more willing to challenge convention.

Young golfers are inspired.

Young golfers like Akshay Bhatia, Cole Hammer, and Matthew Wolff have already begun to make their mark on the sport, inspired by DeChambeau's innovative approach.

De Chambeau's Revolution

The future of golf is bright.

The future of golf is bright, with a new generation of golfers who are passionate, talented, and committed to pushing the boundaries of what is possible.

A New Era of Innovation

DeChambeau's influence has ushered in a new era of innovation in golf, an era that promises to be more exciting, more unpredictable, and more transformative than ever before.

By inspiring a new generation of golfers, DeChambeau is helping to ensure that golf remains vibrant, dynamic,

De Chambeau's Revolution

and relevant—a sport that continues to evolve and thrive for generations to come.

CHAPTER 10 : THE EVOLUTION OF GOLF:

Golf has undergone a remarkable evolution over the centuries, transforming from a humble Scottish pastime to a global sport played by millions.

From Scotland to the World

Golf's origins can be traced back to Scotland in the 15th century, where it was played by noblemen and commoners alike.

The Early Years

De Chambeau's Revolution

In the early years, golf was a rough and ready sport played on links courses with rudimentary equipment.

The Birth of the Modern Game

The modern game of golf began to take shape in the 19th century with the establishment of the first golf clubs and the development of standardised rules.

The Golden Age of Golf

The early 20th century is often referred to as the Golden Age of golf, with legendary players like Bobby Jones and Ben Hogan dominating the sport.

The Technological Revolution

De Chambeau's Revolution

The latter half of the 20th century saw a technological revolution in golf, with advances in equipment, training methods, and course design.

The Modern Game

Today's golf is a high-tech, global sport played by millions of people around the world.

DeChambeau's Impact

Bryson DeChambeau's innovative approach has accelerated golf's evolution, pushing the boundaries of what is possible and inspiring a new generation of golfers.

De Chambeau's Revolution

By understanding golf's evolution, we can appreciate the sport's rich history and exciting future and recognise the role that innovators like DeChambeau have played in shaping the game we know today.

10.1: A Lasting Impact

Bryson DeChambeau's innovative approach to golf has already had a significant impact on the sport, but its long-term effects will be even more profound.

Changing the way players think

De Chambeau's Revolution

DeChambeau's approach has changed the way players think about the game, encouraging them to be more analytical and experimental.

Equipment Innovation

DeChambeau's work with equipment manufacturers has driven innovation, leading to the development of new technologies and training methods.

Course Design Evolution

DeChambeau's approach has also influenced course design, with architects creating more challenging and strategic layouts that reward creative play.

De Chambeau's Revolution

Growing the Game

DeChambeau's influence has helped grow the game, attracting new players and fans who are drawn to his innovative approach.

Creating a New Generation of Innovators

DeChambeau's legacy will be a new generation of innovators who will continue to push the boundaries of what is possible in golf.

A Lasting Impact on the Sport

De Chambeau's Revolution

DeChambeau's approach has had a lasting impact on the sport, changing the way players think, equipment is designed, courses are built, and the game is played.

By examining the long-term effects of DeChambeau's approach, we can gain a deeper understanding of his influence on the sport and the exciting possibilities that lie ahead.

CHAPTER 11: BEYOND THE FAIRWAY

Bryson DeChambeau's life outside the golf course is just as fascinating as his career on it.

De Chambeau's Revolution

Family and upbringing

DeChambeau was raised in a tight-knit family and has spoken publicly about the importance of his parents and siblings in supporting his golf career.

Interests and Hobbies

Away from golf, DeChambeau enjoys reading, working out, and exploring new places.

Philanthropy and Giving Back

DeChambeau is committed to giving back, supporting various charitable causes, and using his platform to make a positive impact.

Friendships and relationships

De Chambeau's Revolution

DeChambeau has formed close friendships with fellow golfers and celebrities and has been linked to several high-profile relationships.

Personal growth and self-care

DeChambeau prioritises personal growth and self-care, recognising the importance of mental and emotional well-being in achieving success.

The Private Side of a Public Figure

Despite his fame and success, DeChambeau values his privacy and keeps certain aspects of his life out of the spotlight.

By exploring DeChambeau's life outside the golf course, we gain a more complete understanding of this fascinating and complex individual.

This chapter could provide a unique perspective on DeChambeau's life, highlighting aspects that may not be well-known to the public.

CONCLUSION

Bryson DeChambeau's innovative approach to golf has sparked a revolution that will be remembered for generations to come.

A look back

DeChambeau's journey has been marked by milestones and achievements that have inspired a new generation of golfers.

A Glance Forward

As we look to the future, it's clear that DeChambeau's influence will continue to shape the sport.

Lasting Impact

DeChambeau's legacy will be a permanent shift in the way golfers think, train, and compete.

De Chambeau's Revolution

Continuing Innovation

DeChambeau's innovative spirit will inspire future generations to continue pushing the boundaries of what is possible.

Growing the Game

DeChambeau's influence has helped grow the game, attracting new players and fans who are drawn to his exciting and dynamic approach.

Cementing a Legacy

DeChambeau's legacy is already cemented, but his continued innovation and success will only add to his impact on the sport.

By examining DeChambeau's legacy, we can gain a deeper understanding of his influence on the sport and the exciting possibilities that lie ahead.

www.ingramcontent.com/pod-product-compliance
Lightning Source LLC
Chambersburg PA
CBHW071955210526
45479CB00003B/954